Polymyositis: Causes, Tests and Treatments

John Hewitt MA

Editor in Chief: James Greenspan *MD*

© 2011 John Hewitt, MA, James Greenspan

All Rights Reserved worldwide under the Berne Convention. May not be copied or distributed without prior written permission by the publisher. If you have this book or an electronic document and didn't pay for it, then the author didn't get a fair share. Please consider paying for your copy by purchasing it at <u>any bookstore or online retailer</u>. Thank you!

Printed in the United States of America

ISBN 9781468106046

Contents

One: What is Polymyositis? 4
Two: Why do You Get Polymyositis? 7
Three: Common symptoms for Polymyositis 10
Four: How can I know if I have Polymyositis? 14
Five: Medical treatment 20
Six: Side-effects of medical treatment 27
Seven: Self help treatment 32
A Genetics Primer 38
Glossary of Medical Terms 80
Appendix A: Internet Resources / Further Reading 98

[3]

One: What is Polymyositis?

Polymyositis (PM) is an inflammatory muscle disease that causes weakness and swelling of the skeletal muscles, which control movement.

Explains why I can't move during flare up. and pain and weakness.

The condition usually develops with general weakness and muscle pain and then progresses to a stage where muscle pain becomes so severe that you may be unable to move or walk. You may even be unable to raise your arms above your head due to the pain. If it affects your leg muscles, it can grow so severe that you may fall while walking. You may be unable to walk or do any physical activity involving your shoulder, neck, or hip muscles. The condition is usually prevalent in the elderly and rarely occurs in young people. Women are more often affected by it than men.

White blood cells are part of the defense system of our body. But sometimes, they start acting strangely. They attack the lining of the muscles and start to destroy them, causing the muscular weakness associated with polymyositis. No one knows exactly why the white blood cells start acting this way all of a sudden, although doctors believe this may be because of genetic factor, or certain infections, which leaves behind infection in the body, causing the white blood cells to stay active.

Shingles? Triggered?

The symptoms of Polymyositis develop gradually over three to six months. Diagnosis of this condition is a difficult task because you may see no clear symptoms while the disease progresses to a severe level. Most patients tend to ignore weak muscular pain or weakness, thinking it is a minor condition - the "aches and pains" of getting older. Another difficulty in diagnosing this condition is that it is often a result of certain other diseases such as infections by viruses. Initially, the virus may be blamed for your symptoms.

You will have to go through a number of tests for the initial disease. After your doctor confirms that you have polymyositis, you will again have to go through a number of tests. This is because polymyositis causes many other problems within your body, including: throat problems or lung problems which include dry cough and labored breathing. You may have difficulty in swallowing or eating which eventually becomes so severe that you can't speak properly. Your heart may be affected by polymyositis and in the most severe case you may suffer from a cardiac arrest.

If you are suffering from this condition, you may experience periods of severe and then slight symptoms. At times, the condition may be so severe that you are unable to

FLARE UP TIME
OMH? [6]

walk or do your daily physical activities. At other times, it may subside to slight pain in the muscles and you may feel a dramatic improvement. But if you feel that type of improvement with polymyositis, it is only temporary and the pain will likely return with a vengeance. You should not stop taking any prescribed medication if you see any temporary improvement; if you want to reduce the dosage of your medication, you should consult with your doctor first.

The muscles which are most often affected in polymyositis are the ones close to the trunk, mainly the muscles of your neck, upper arms, shoulders, thighs, and hips.

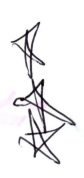

Two: Why do You Get Polymyositis?

Usually, women are more at risk of getting polymyositis than men with an approximate 2:1 ratio. Also, the disease is known to be more common among the elderly than the young. However, this doesn't mean that young people don't get polymyositis. There have been rare cases when some patients acquired the disease during their mid-childhood years. But in most cases, people acquire this disease in their forties.

Many other diseases share symptoms with polymyositis. Diseases such as polymyalgia rheumatica are also marked with muscular fatigue and pain. And like polymyalgia rheumatica, there is no certain cause for polymyositis.

Polymyositis shares many characteristics with autoimmune diseases, in which the immune system attacks normal body tissues. Normally, the immune system protects the body against foreign harmful substances, such as viruses and bacteria. In Polymyositis, an unknown cause acts as a trigger for the immune system to produce autoantibodies that attack the normal body tissues. Some doctors say that the condition is acquired genetically. This means that if you suffer from polymyositis, this is because the genes for this disease were transferred to you by your parents. This may be because one or both of your parents also suffered from this disease or at least had it in their genes.

Other doctors suggest that polymyositis usually occurs only after some other infection or disease has weakened or disturbed the body's immune system. White blood cells are the cells which constitute the defense system of our body and resist any infections. Some diseases such as bacterial infections may cause these cells to act in such a way that they attack the body itself, attacking the lining of certain muscles. For example, diseases which cause inflammation raise the level of muscle enzymes in the body. White blood cells consider that a threat to the body and start attacking the muscles. This, too, can cause polymyositis. And this is why often the treatment of polymyositis includes the use of medication to reduce the level of muscle enzymes in the body.

Since the cause of this disease is unknown, doctors will check your medical history to see if you suffer from any other diseases. This is because polymyositis is also thought to be a result of bacterial and viral infections and through their diagnosis, it will become easier for the doctor to diagnose and treat polymyositis. You should also tell your doctor about any recent infections or if you have had an allergic reaction to food recently.

Three: Common symptoms for Polymyositis

Symptoms of polymyositis appear are slowly progressive and may also fluctuate from week to week or month to month.

If you think you are suffering from polymyositis, check the following symptoms. If you think you have polymyositis, contact your doctor as soon as possible:

- Morning stiffness. When you wake up in the morning, your muscles might be so stiff that moving them or doing anything physical is painful. Stiffness in the muscles may decrease as the day progresses but is most severe in the mornings or after relaxation. Normally, towards the evening, the muscle stiffness is nearly gone entirely and you may be able to work as normal.

- Muscular pain in neck, shoulders, hips, and thighs. Typically, polymyositis pain starts in the hip muscles, leading to difficulty in rising from a seated position and ascending stairs. Neck muscles, shoulders muscles and upper arm muscles may be also affected. The pain in the upper arms and shoulders might get so severe at times that you are unable to raise your arms above your shoulders.

- **Anorexia.** Anorexia is a disorder causing loss of appetite. This results in malnutrition and leads to weight loss. Anorexia is among the common symptoms of polymyositis. Anorexia in patients with polymyositis is caused by difficult swallowing (dysphagia) and depression. Both dysphagia and depression are common in polymyositis patients.

- **Lung problems.** Lung problems are common among polymyositis patients. About 15 to 30 percent of polymyositis patients suffer from lung diseases, such as interstitial lung disease (ILD). If you suffer from dry cough or experience difficulty in breathing, this most likely means that you are also suffering from lung problems associated with polymyositis. If you feel that you are experiencing any of these symptoms, you should contact a pulmonary specialist who will prescribe you the right medicine to suppress them.

- **Cardiac / heart problems.** Polymyositis patients also tend to suffer from heart problems, such as heart failure and irregular heart beating (arrhythmias).

Severe polymyositis can affect the heart muscle, leading to cardiomyopathy and heart failure. You should see a cardiologist if you face any heart-related problems, such as fatigue, difficult breathing and swelling of the legs and feet.

- The muscles of the pharynx and esophagus may be affected. This results in difficulty swallowing (dysphagia) which occurs in 30% of patients with polymyositis. When you feel that swallowing becomes difficult, contact your doctor for the right medicine. If you leave it untreated, foods or liquids, including saliva will be aspirated into your lungs (aspiration), which can lead inflammation of the lungs (pneumonia). Also, the muscles of the larynx may be affected leading to difficulty in speaking (dysarthria).
- Constipation. Patients of Polymyositis often also suffer from constipation.
- Arthralgia. In this condition, the patient suffers from inflamed and swollen joints.
- Rough skin or slight wounds on the palm and inner side of the fingers. This condition is usually termed 'Mechanic's hands.'
- Abdominal swelling and nose bleeds

may be present.

Four: How can I know if I have Polymyositis?

Polymyositis is not an easy disease to diagnose. This is mostly because no definite reason is known for the cause of this disease which leads to a number of tests which have to be conducted to diagnose you. Another huge difficulty in diagnosing polymyositis is that this disease slowly progresses within your body. You won't be aware of it while it progresses and there won't be any serious symptoms to hint that there is a problem. The disease takes three to six months to develop. And only when it has fully developed, then you may experience the full range of symptoms.

When you go to your doctor for a polymyositis diagnosis, your doctor will take your detailed medical history and will check for a number of other diseases which accompany polymyositis such as heart and lung complications. To diagnose the related diseases, you will have to undergo a number of medical tests.

Your doctor will initially ask to take basic medical tests such as different blood tests to determine the level of muscle enzymes. Increased muscle enzymes level can indicate muscle damage. He may also ask you to get an

Creatine Kinase very high prior to last April 2023 Flare Up.

MRI or muscle testing such as electromyography. This test is also used to determine muscle biopsy sites. In polymyositis, a muscle biopsy typically shows inflamed and dead muscle cells (necrosis).

Different muscle strength tests are used to check your muscle strength. If your muscles indicate weakness, there is a high probability that you have polymyositis. One example of such a test is range-of-motion. This refers to the distance and direction a joint can move normally. If this test indicates that the joint can't move normally to the full possible distance and direction, this may indicate the presence of polymyositis.

The blood tests which are usually prescribed for polymyositis are used to check the level of muscle enzymes. Enzymes are a part of body which help in the carrying out of chemical reactions. The diagnosis of polymyositis is done by checking the level of creatine kinase, an enzyme. If you are suffering from polymyositis, the level of this enzyme in your body will be five to 50 times higher than normal. This high level of muscle enzyme indicates muscle damage; that is what makes your muscles feel weak. The levels of other enzymes such as lactate dehydrogenase, alanine aminotransferase, aldolase and aspartate aminotransferase are also checked. They are usually higher than normal in polymyositis patients.

Other tests include electrical tests which are used to indicate any abnormality in muscles or nerves. Examples are electromyography (EMG) and nerve conduction velocity tests.

Electro-diagnosis:

Electromyography (EMG) is a kind of electrical test used to diagnose different diseases. It can be a very helpful tool in diagnosing a patient with polymyositis. Electro-diagnosis checks muscles for the signs of polymyositis. A thin needle is inserted into the muscle to be tested. If the test results indicate that muscles are weak or if any other of the related signs of polymyositis are seen in the muscles such as an abnormality in the nerves that control the muscles, it is very likely that you are suffering from the condition. But it is not completely foolproof. It simply confirms the symptoms of polymyositis related to muscles. Sometimes, other diseases also show similar test results for electro-diagnosis and this test alone cannot confirm whether or not you have polymyositis.

Polymyositis is not an isolated disease. Most of the time, you get polymyositis due to the infection caused by another disease or after another disease leaves your body weaker. Also, once you have polymyositis, you will also be at a high risk of suffering from a number of other diseases related to lungs, throat and heart. Your doctor may ask you to undergo different tests so that you can be sure that you are not suffering from any of related diseases. These tests are called differential diagnosis tests and may include diagnosis for:

- Muscular dystrophy: This is a disease in which muscles grow weak and muscle tissue is lost.
- Endocrine Myopathy: In this disease, striated muscles are affected by diseases of the endocrine system, such as thyroid, parathyroid, suprarenal and pituitary glands.
- HIV associated myopathy:
- Acute inflammatory Demyelinating Polyneuropathy: This disease affects the nerves that control the muscles.
- Chronic inflammatory Demyelinating Polyneuropathy: This disease has same symptoms as acute inflammatory demyelinating polyneuropathy but it is more long-term.

- **HIV associated neuromuscular disease:** This includes a range of diseases which are caused by HIV.
- **Amyotrophic Lateral Sclerosis:** This disease is related to neuron disorders. Symptoms are severe weakness of muscles which may lead to failure of muscles. It may also cause respiratory problems and can cause death.
- **Inclusion body myositis:** This disease severely effects and damages the muscles of arms and legs.
- **Biochemical muscle disease**

Other tests which are usually advised for a polymyositis patient are:

- **Thyroid Function tests:** This is a term used for a number of blood tests which are used to check whether the thyroid is working properly.
- **Complete blood count:** CBC tests are used to get information about the cells in a patient's blood.
- **ANA:** The Antinuclear Antibody test. This test is used to detect autoantibodies.

Positive results may indicate that the defense system of the body is functioning abnormally.

- **Urea/Electrolytes**, particularly K+: This test is usually used to check the functioning of the kidney.

- **Creatinine kinase (CK)**: This test is used to check the level of creatinine kinase in the muscles. CK is a muscle enzyme and high levels of CK in the muscles damages them.

- **Anti Jo-1 antibodies**: They are a type of anti-nuclear antibodies. High level of anti Jo-1 antibodies may indicate arthritis and interstitial lung disease which are common associations of polymyositis.

Five: Medical treatment

Polymyositis treatments can vary. A number of drugs and therapies are used to treat this condition. A common treatment that is often prescribed to polymyositis patients is the use of corticosteroids. These are a type of steroid which is used to control inflammation and reduce the production of antibodies in the body. Antibodies are proteins which are a part of the body's defensive mechanism. But when you suffer from polymyositis, the immune system of the body malfunctions and there may be an abnormal production of antibodies. This high level of antibodies attacks the muscles and weakens them. To prevent this abnormal production, your doctor prescribes you corticosteroids.

The other method of treating antibodies is therapy through medicine. Following are the different therapies that may be effective against antibodies.

Intravenous immunoglobulin (IVIg):

In this method of treatment, antibodies and immunoglobulin from healthy donors are taken. High doses of these are then given to the polymyositis patient. The result is that these high doses block the antibodies in your own body that are harming your muscle linings. But treatment with intravenous immunoglobulin is only short-term.

Immunosuppressive Therapy:

If you are suffering from polymyositis, there is a high chance that you are also suffering from a skin disease with symptoms such as skin rashes. Having polymyositis also means that you are very likely to suffer from different lung diseases. Immunosuppressive therapy is used to cure these problems. It is also used when you witness no improvement even after using corticosteroids for four continuous weeks. In this therapy, a drug named tacrolimuc (Prograf) is used. Usually this drug is used as a transplant rejection drug. Immunosuppressive agents are fairly effective in most cases, but may be needed as a life-long treatment.

Polymyositis and its symptoms of muscular weakness are caused mainly because of the immune disorder in which white blood cells mistake body parts for being infected segments and then attack them. Immunosuppressive agents are quite impressive and effective in that they suppress the response of white blood cells so that they don't attack the muscles as much.

The medicinal treatment for polymyositis typically comprises of:

- The use of corticosteroids. The most commonly used corticosteroid is prednisone. Prednisone is the most basic and common medicine that is prescribed to polymyositis patients. It is usually helpful in reducing the inflammation or swelling of muscles. If you are suffering from the condition, your doctor will recommend you use this medicine. The dose is 1 mg per day either as a single dose or as divided doses throughout the day. This relatively high dose is continued for about four to eight weeks and meanwhile, your doctor keeps checking the CK levels. Once the CK levels return to normal, which is usually no later than eight weeks, your doctor will start reducing the dose. The dose is reduced by 5 - 10 mg every month until the minimum dose needed to control CK levels is found.

- Immunosuppressive agents. These agents are prescribed by the doctor in two cases: if you are using corticosteroids to treat polymyositis and these steroids are not working, or if you are suffering from the side-effects of these.

Methotrexate is an immunosuppressive agent that is commonly prescribed. Azathioprine is also an oft-used immunosuppressive agent.

- When you are suffering from polymyositis, you are also very likely to suffer from different lung diseases. In most cases, an effective cure for the lung problems associated with polymyositis is cyclophosphamide.

Polymyositis is a serious condition. It can cause severe health problems and even death if it's not properly treated. However, if you take proper care, get it diagnosed timely and follow the right treatments, together with the right lifestyle and dietary habits, you can live a normal, healthy life. Since this condition affects the body in many different ways, you may have to consult the following specialists for effective treatment:

- Neuropsychologist (For the adverse effects of polymyositis on mental health. The use of steroids can induce mental health problems and you may end up feeling depressed or suffering from some other mental condition. To overcome these problems, you should make routine visit to a neuropsychologist so that your mental health is not disturbed. The neuropsychologist will help you identify how your mental health is being affected and will advise you how to treat your condition.)

- Cardiologists (Cardiologist will help you avoid or treat heart problems which are often faced by polymyositis patients. If polymyositis related heart problems are not treated properly and in time, you may be risking a heart attack. To avoid such a severe outcome, include a trip to a cardiologist once a month in your routine.)

- Pulmonologist (To effectively cure lung problems. Typical lung problems associated with polymyositis are dry cough and a difficulty in breathing. If you face difficulty in breathing you should immediately contact a pulmonary specialist because that could indicate a serious lung problem.)

- Rheumatologists (A rheumatologist will help you if you suffer from arthritis, a condition in which your joints become inflamed and swollen. If you are suffering from polymyositis, there is a high chance that you have also acquired arthritis.)

- Speech therapists (To help you if you have swallowing difficulties. Often, the weakness and pain in the muscles makes eating, chewing, swallowing and speaking very painful. If this is left untreated, this can lead to severe symptoms where even speaking causes a lot of pain and becomes difficult. If you face this, a speech therapist will tell you about different exercises that will enable you to overcome the speech problems.)

- Physical therapists (To help you get over the muscular weakness through physical therapy. Exercise is a must activity for polymyositis patients. If you don't exercise, you won't be able to counter the disease effectively. Contact a physical therapist to know which exercises are good for you and which are not. Some exercises which involve severe physical exertion are often not a good fit for polymyositis patients.)

As a polymyositis patient, you should visit your doctor every two to three weeks for different tests. These tests will check your enzyme levels and see if they are normal and will also check your muscle strength to confirm that the disease is not progressing. Once you get stable and the disease stops progressing, this means you are improving and you can schedule a visit with your doctor once in a month. You should also get your weight checked monthly so that it doesn't register either an abnormal weight loss or weight gain. An abnormal weight loss can be due to the fact that your muscles are weakening. Abnormal weight gain can be a result of the long-term use of corticosteroids.

↳ longer than 30 days
Generally only Rx'd for 1-2 weeks
for acute symptoms (bag ked)

Six: Side-effects of medical treatment

Corticosteroids are the most commonly used steroids used for the medical treatment of polymyositis. The use of steroids has a number of side-effects.

Following are the possible side-effects of using steroids in high doses:

- Immune system problems. The use of steroids adversely affects the immune system. Due to the weakening of immune system, you may run a high chance of acquiring many other diseases apart from polymyositis itself.
- Obesity. Another common characteristic of corticosteroids usage is that they increase your appetite and you tend to eat more. This often results in a weight gain and makes some people obese. It also leads to a puffiness of the face (moon face).
- Muscle weakness. Prednisone is the most commonly used corticosteroid. It stops the progress of the disease and is quite effective in curing it. But as a side-effect, it also causes muscle

weakness.

- **Skin problems**. High-dose corticosteroids usage can lead to a sensitive thin skin which easily becomes bruised.

- **High blood pressure** and **diabetes**. Patients who have a history of blood pressure problems or diabetes should use corticosteroids very carefully. This is because corticosteroids tend to increase blood pressure and can make diabetes worse. If you have diabetes or if anyone in your family has diabetes, then there is a high chance that steroid use will cause some problems for you. Your doctor can prescribe medication to prevent the steroids from worsening your diabetes.

- **Osteoporosis** is another side-effect of steroids. Osteoporosis means thinning of bones. If you are 65 or older, then you have a very high risk of acquiring osteoporosis. In addition, if you have a history of bone fractures which suggests that you have weak bones, you are very vulnerable to this condition. Normally, the disease is preventable and controllable; if it is diagnosed at the right time and adequately treated, it won't be dangerous at all. Your doctor will simply prescribe you some drug that you will have to use along with the steroids to counter the side-effects. You can get the strength of your bones checked through a DEXA scan.

- **Abruptly stopping** the usage of corticosteroids can also lead to different adverse effects. These include vomiting, nausea and blood pressure problems. Therefore, you should withdraw from corticosteroids gradually and with the advice of your doctor. If while reducing the dose and trying to withdraw you experience any of these side effects, you should immediately report them to your doctor.

- Another important medication used for the treatment of polymyositis is immunosuppressive agents. These agents have a number of side-effects. Their use can cause different liver and bone-marrow problems. If you are using these medications together with the corticosteroids for the treatment of your polymyositis, you should regularly get your blood monitored.

- The use of immunosuppressive agents can also lead to a number of lung-related diseases. Consult your doctor regularly while taking such agents and use some drug such as cyclosporine to avoid such side-effects if your doctor suggests.

- Steroids can also cause eye-problems. In some severe cases, prolonged use of corticosteroids can cause cataracts.

- Steroids may cause gastrointestinal bleeding. Prolonged use can also cause stomach ulcers. If you feel any abdominal pains during steroid use, this means that either of the two cases could be true. Immediately consult your doctor if you experience abdominal pain while taking steroids.

- The use of corticosteroids is normally a long-term treatment and is generally effective in treating polymyositis and helping a patient live normal life. But a huge side-effect of long-term usage of this steroid is that your body grows dependent on the steroids; it stops producing the right amount of hormones needed, especially hormones produced by adrenal glands, and becomes dependent upon steroids to fulfill the need. So when you stop using corticosteroid, your body may not produce the right amounts of hormones. If you are scheduled for surgery or an operation, you should tell your doctor about your steroids use because during surgery or operation, high levels of hormones may be needed to counteract the effects of the steroid use.

- Long-term dose of corticosteroids can also cause night sweats, facial hair growth and upset stomach. It can lead to sensitive emotions and depression.

- Prednisone can cause insomnia. Sleeplessness can enhance your feeling of physical weakness. It can lead to weak mental health which triggers negative thoughts, even suicidal thoughts. Therefore, it's vital for a polymyositis patient to regularly visit a neuropsychologist so that if he acquired any mental health issues, the neurologist diagnoses them timely and suggests a cure for it.

Seven: Self help treatment

Medical treatment is most commonly used to cure polymyositis. And it is quite effective in treating the disease. But the problem with medical treatment is that it has a number of side-effects. And these side-effects appear during the time you are taking the drugs and even after that in the form of weakness.

There is another way of treating polymyositis. It is not entirely effective but it can ensure one thing: that you face minimal side-effects of the medical treatment. Not only that, this way also helps you recover sooner and in a far better way. A modified diet and more healthy working and living habits means that you can defeat polymyositis much more successfully. Here is a list of non-medicinal methods and the details of how to use them:

- **Exercise:**

    If you are suffering from polymyositis, it is highly recommended that you take up exercise. If you have an exercise routine, continue what you have been doing. If you don't, you should immediately maintain a daily exercise routine after you consult with your doctor. The exercise does not need to be very tough or physically trying. In fact, if you feel that you can't do exercises which involve physical exertion, then try low impact exercise like walking. This is an exercise which is possible for nearly everyone. Just set a routine, preferably in the morning, to take a walk or a mile or two. This will greatly enhance your health. You may also consult your doctor or physical therapist about your exercise routine. They may suggest appropriate exercises that can fit in with your lifestyle and physical limitations. You must be careful not to overdo it. Sometimes, too rigorous exercise can lead to adverse effects rather than benefitting you.

Normally, you will be asked by your doctor to take up light gym exercises. Such exercises help you get muscle mass and overcome muscle weakness.

- **Diet:**

    If you are suffering of polymyositis,

it is very important that you maintain a healthy diet and eat or drink only such foods which do no harm during polymyositis.

For example, if polymyositis has affected your tongue or throat muscles, you need to adjust your diet so that you eat food which does not affect your throat muscles much. Consult with a nutritionist and speech therapist who will tell you which food is okay for you to take and which will cause you problems.

A nutritionist can also help you develop a diet plan which suits your condition. Since the cause of polymyositis is not known, some doctors think that it may be an outcome of an unbalanced diet or having something in your diet which causes certain allergies and then leads to polymyositis. If you get help from a nutritionist, he will assess your dietary habits and will help you discover which foods are not good for you. He will let you find out your food intolerances and allergies and will lay out a food plan for out which rules out foods to which your body reacts adversely. This will not only save you from getting other harmful diseases, it will also help you to recover from polymyositis.

※ High Protein Diet ※

Generally, a high-protein diet is very good for you if you are suffering from polymyositis. Also, your diet should also provide sufficient amounts of calcium to your body. For this purpose, you can include orange juice, skimmed and low-fat milk, low-fat sugarless yogurt and salmon in your diet. Apart from these, if you still feel weakness due to steroids intake, you should start taking calcium supplements with the advice of your doctor. These supplements have barely any side effects. Calcium is essential for you as a polymyositis patient because the steroids you take can greatly harm your bones and make them weak. And calcium intake is the best way to counter such a side-effect.

Processed food is also not very healthy for a polymyositis patient. You should avoid it as much as you can because patients who avoid processed food have been found to recover sooner from polymyositis than those who have processed food in their diet.

You should include zinc, selenium and vitamin A, C and E supplements to your diet. They are also good for polymyositis patients.

- **Work habits:**

Polymyositis is a disease that cannot be fully cured. At most, you can control it and stop it from progressing. But that needs very strong determination. If you want to control your polymyositis, you have to work hard for it. You have to take up exercise, dietary control, get regular check-ups, and see your doctor and therapists regularly. The slightest carelessness leads you straight to point zero and dump all improvement made through treatment. If you really want to benefit from treatment, you have to manage every single day in a way that suits your condition and does not affect it adversely. A number of patients have shown significant improvement in their polymyositis - some of them have controlled it and they lead very normal and healthy lives. But for that, they strive hard. They see speech therapists and do speech exercises regularly if they have problems with swallowing. They do extensive physical exercises so that the weakness caused by polymyositis is balanced by the muscle mass created from exercising. They get frequent check-ups to confirm that their enzyme levels are normal.

So if you have polymyositis and if you wish to battle with it and defeat it, revamp your living style today. You have to rearrange everything, review your habits and organize your days and nights carefully.

A Genetics Primer

Although genetics can't cure any disease, understanding how and why genetic defects occur can help stop the gene from transmitting from parent to child.

Genetics (from Ancient Greek γενετικός genetikos, "genitive" and that from γένεσις genesis, "origin"[1][2][3]), a discipline of biology, is the science of genes, heredity, and variation in living organisms.[4][5] The fact that living things inherit traits from their parents has been used since prehistoric times to improve crop plants and animals through selective breeding. However, the modern science of genetics, which seeks to understand the process of inheritance, only began with the work of Gregor Mendel in the mid-19th century.[6] Although he did not know the physical basis for heredity, Mendel observed that organisms inherit traits via discrete units of inheritance, which are now called genes.

Genes correspond to regions within DNA, a molecule composed of a chain of four different types of nucleotides-the sequence of these nucleotides is the genetic information organisms inherit. DNA naturally occurs in a double stranded form, with nucleotides on each strand complementary to each other. Each strand can act as a template for creating a new partner strand-this is the physical method for making copies of genes that can be inherited.

The sequence of nucleotides in a gene is translated by cells to produce a chain of amino acids, creating proteins-the order of amino acids in a protein corresponds to the order of nucleotides in the gene. This relationship between nucleotide sequence and amino acid sequence is known as the genetic code. The amino acids in a protein determine how it folds into a three-dimensional shape; this structure is, in turn, responsible for the protein's function. Proteins carry out almost all the functions needed for cells to live. A change to the DNA in a gene can change a protein's amino acids, changing its shape and function: this can have a dramatic effect in the cell and on the organism as a whole.

Although genetics plays a large role in the appearance and behavior of organisms, it is the combination of genetics with what an organism experiences that determines the ultimate outcome. For example, while genes play a role in determining an organism's size, the nutrition and other conditions it experiences after inception also have a large effect.

History of genetics

DNA is the molecular basis for inheritance. Each strand of DNA is a chain of nucleotides, matching each other in the center to form what look like rungs on a twisted ladder.

Although the science of genetics began with the

applied and theoretical work of Gregor Mendel in the mid-19th century, other theories of inheritance preceded Mendel. A popular theory during Mendel's time was the concept of blending inheritance: the idea that individuals inherit a smooth blend of traits from their parents. Mendel's work disproved this, showing that traits are composed of combinations of distinct genes rather than a continuous blend. Another theory that had some support at that time was the inheritance of acquired characteristics: the belief that individuals inherit traits strengthened by their parents. This theory (commonly associated with Jean-Baptiste Lamarck) is now known to be wrong-the experiences of individuals do not affect the genes they pass to their children.[7] Other theories included the pangenesis of Charles Darwin (which had both acquired and inherited aspects) and Francis Galton's reformulation of pangenesis as both particulate and inherited.[8]

Mendelian and classical genetics

The modern science of genetics traces its roots to Gregor Johann Mendel, a German-Czech Augustinian monk and scientist who studied the nature of inheritance in plants. In his paper "Versuche über Pflanzenhybriden" ("Experiments on Plant Hybridization"), presented in 1865 to the Natur forschender Verein (Society for Research in

Nature) in Brünn, Mendel traced the inheritance patterns of certain traits in pea plants and described them mathematically.[9] Although this pattern of inheritance could only be observed for a few traits, Mendel's work suggested that heredity was particulate, not acquired, and that the inheritance patterns of many traits could be explained through simple rules and ratios.

The importance of Mendel's work did not gain wide understanding until the 1890s, after his death, when other scientists working on similar problems re-discovered his research. William Bateson, a proponent of Mendel's work, coined the word genetics in 1905.[10][11] (The adjective genetic, derived from the Greek word genesis-γένεσις, "origin" and that from the word genno-γεννώ, "to give birth", predates the noun and was first used in a biological sense in 1860.)[12] Bateson popularized the usage of the word genetics to describe the study of inheritance in his inaugural address to the Third International Conference on Plant Hybridization in London, England, in 1906.[13]

After the rediscovery of Mendel's work, scientists tried to determine which molecules in the cell were responsible for inheritance. In 1910, Thomas Hunt Morgan argued that genes are on chromosomes, based on observations of a sex-linked white eye mutation in fruit flies.[14] In 1913, his student Alfred Sturtevant used the phenomenon of genetic linkage to show that genes are arranged linearly on the chromosome.[15]

Morgan's observation of sex-linked inheritance of a mutation causing white eyes in Drosophila led him to the hypothesis that genes are located upon chromosomes.

Molecular Genetics

Although genes were known to exist on chromosomes, chromosomes are composed of both protein and DNA-scientists did not know which of these is responsible for inheritance. In 1928, Frederick Griffith discovered the phenomenon of transformation (see Griffith's experiment): dead bacteria could transfer genetic material to "transform" other still-living bacteria. Sixteen years later, in 1944, Oswald Theodore Avery, Colin McLeod and Maclyn McCarty identified the molecule responsible for transformation as DNA.[16] The Hershey-Chase experiment in 1952 also showed that DNA (rather than protein) is the genetic material of the viruses that infect bacteria, providing further evidence that DNA is the molecule responsible for inheritance.[17]

James D. Watson and Francis Crick determined the structure of DNA in 1953, using the X-ray crystallography work of Rosalind Franklin and Maurice Wilkins that indicated

[43]

DNA had a helical structure (i.e., shaped like a corkscrew).[18][19] Their double-helix model had two strands of DNA with the nucleotides pointing inward, each matching a complementary nucleotide on the other strand to form what looks like rungs on a twisted ladder.[20] This structure showed that genetic information exists in the sequence of nucleotides on each strand of DNA. The structure also suggested a simple method for duplication: if the strands are separated, new partner strands can be reconstructed for each based on the sequence of the old strand.

Although the structure of DNA showed how inheritance works, it was still not known how DNA influences the behavior of cells. In the following years, scientists tried to understand how DNA controls the process of protein production. It was discovered that the cell uses DNA as a template to create matching messenger RNA (a molecule with nucleotides, very similar to DNA). The nucleotide sequence of a messenger RNA is used to create an amino acid sequence in protein; this translation between nucleotide and amino acid sequences is known as the genetic code.

With this molecular understanding of inheritance, an explosion of research became possible. One important development was chain-termination DNA sequencing in 1977 by Frederick Sanger. This technology allows scientists to read the nucleotide sequence of a DNA molecule.[21] In 1983, Kary Banks Mullis developed the polymerase chain reaction, providing a quick way to isolate and amplify a specific section of a DNA from a mixture.[22] Through the pooled efforts of the Human Genome Project and the parallel private effort by Celera Genomics, these and other techniques culminated in the sequencing of the human genome in 2003.[23]

Mendelian Inheritance

At its most fundamental level, inheritance in organisms occurs by means of discrete traits, called genes.[24] This property was first observed by Gregor Mendel, who studied the segregation of heritable traits in pea plants.[9][25] In his experiments studying the trait for flower color, Mendel observed that the flowers of each pea plant were either purple or white-but never an intermediate between the two colors. These different, discrete versions of the same gene are called alleles.

In the case of pea, which is a diploid species, each individual plant has two alleles of each gene, one allele inherited from each parent.[26] Many species, including humans, have this pattern of inheritance. Diploid organisms with two copies of the same allele of a given gene are called homozygous at that gene locus, while organisms with two different alleles of a given gene are called heterozygous.

The set of alleles for a given organism is called its genotype, while the observable traits of the organism are called its phenotype. When organisms are heterozygous at a gene, often one allele is called dominant as its qualities dominate the phenotype of the organism, while the other allele is called recessive as its qualities recede and are not observed. Some alleles do not have complete dominance and instead have incomplete dominance by expressing an intermediate phenotype, or codominance by expressing both alleles at once.[27]

When a pair of organisms reproduce sexually, their offspring randomly inherit one of the two alleles from each parent. These observations of discrete inheritance and the segregation of alleles are collectively known as Mendel's first law or the Law of Segregation.

Geneticists use diagrams and symbols to describe inheritance. A gene is represented by one or a few letters. Often a "+" symbol is used to mark the usual, non-mutant allele for a gene.[28]

In fertilization and breeding experiments (and especially when discussing Mendel's laws) the parents are referred to as the "P" generation and the offspring as the "F1" (first filial) generation. When the F1 offspring mate with each other, the offspring are called the "F2" (second filial) generation. One of the common diagrams used to predict the result of cross-breeding is the Punnett square.

When studying human genetic diseases, geneticists often use pedigree charts to represent the inheritance of traits.[29] These charts map the inheritance of a trait in a family tree.

Interactions of Multiple Genes

Human height is a complex genetic trait. Francis Galton's data from 1889 shows the relationship between offspring height as a function of mean parent height. While correlated, remaining variation in offspring heights indicates environment is also an important factor in this trait.

Organisms have thousands of genes, and in sexually reproducing organisms these genes generally assort independently of each other. This means that the inheritance of an allele for yellow or green pea color is unrelated to the inheritance of alleles for white or purple flowers. This phenomenon, known as "Mendel's second law" or the "Law of independent assortment", means that the alleles of different genes get shuffled between parents to form offspring with many different combinations. (Some genes do not assort independently, demonstrating genetic linkage, a topic discussed later in this chapter.)

Often different genes can interact in a way that influences the same trait. In the Blue-eyed Mary (Omphalodes verna), for example, there exists a gene with alleles that determine the color of flowers: blue or magenta. Another gene, however, controls whether the flowers have color at all or are white. When a plant has two copies of this white allele, its flowers are white-regardless of whether the first gene has blue or magenta alleles. This interaction between genes is called epistasis, with the second gene epistatic to the first.[30]

Many traits are not discrete features (e.g. purple or white flowers) but are instead continuous features (e.g. human height and skin color). These complex traits are products of many genes.[31] The influence of these genes is mediated, to varying degrees, by the environment an organism has experienced. The degree to which an organism's genes contribute to a complex trait is called heritability.[32] Measurement of the heritability of a trait is relative-in a more variable environment, the environment has a bigger influence on the total variation of the trait. For example, human height is a complex trait with a heritability of 89% in the United States. In Nigeria, however, where people experience a more variable access to good nutrition and health care, height has a heritability of only 62%.[33]

DNA and Chromosome

The molecular structure of DNA. Bases pair through the arrangement of hydrogen bonding between the strands.

The molecular basis for genes is deoxyribonucleic acid (DNA). DNA is composed of a chain of nucleotides, of which there are four types: adenine (A), cytosine (C), guanine (G), and thymine (T). Genetic information exists in the sequence of these nucleotides, and genes exist as stretches of sequence along the DNA chain.[34] Viruses are the only exception to this rule-sometimes viruses use the very similar molecule RNA instead of DNA as their genetic material.[35]

DNA normally exists as a double-stranded molecule, coiled into the shape of a double-helix. Each nucleotide in DNA preferentially pairs with its partner nucleotide on the opposite strand: A pairs with T, and C pairs with G. Thus, in its two-stranded form, each strand effectively contains all necessary information, redundant with its partner strand. This structure of DNA is the physical basis for inheritance: DNA replication duplicates the genetic information by splitting the strands and using each strand as a template for synthesis of a new partner strand.[36]

Genes are arranged linearly along long chains of DNA sequence, called chromosomes. In bacteria, each cell usually contains a single circular chromosome, while eukaryotic organisms (including plants and animals) have their DNA arranged in multiple linear chromosomes. These DNA strands are often extremely long; the largest human chromosome, for example, is about 247 million base pairs in length.[37] The DNA of a chromosome is associated with structural proteins that organize, compact, and control access to the DNA, forming a material called chromatin; in eukaryotes, chromatin is usually composed of nucleosomes, segments of DNA wound around cores of histone proteins.[38] The full set of hereditary material in an organism (usually the combined DNA sequences of all chromosomes) is called the genome.

While haploid organisms have only one copy of each chromosome, most animals and many plants are diploid, containing two of each chromosome and thus two copies of every gene.[26] The two alleles for a gene are located on identical loci of sister chromatids, each allele inherited from a different parent.

Walther Flemming's 1882 diagram of eukaryotic cell division. Chromosomes are copied, condensed, and organized. Then, as the cell divides, chromosome copies separate into the daughter cells.

An exception exists in the sex chromosomes, specialized chromosomes many animals have evolved that play a role in determining the sex of an organism.[39] In humans and other mammals, the Y chromosome has very few genes and triggers the development of male sexual characteristics, while the X chromosome is similar to the other chromosomes and contains many genes unrelated to sex determination. Females have two copies of the X chromosome, but males have one Y and only one X chromosome; this difference in X chromosome copy numbers leads to the unusual inheritance patterns of sex-linked disorders.

Asexual Reproduction and Sexual Reproduction

When cells divide, their full genome is copied and each daughter cell inherits one copy. This process, called mitosis, is the simplest form of reproduction and is the basis for asexual reproduction. Asexual reproduction can also occur in multicellular organisms, producing offspring that inherit their genome from a single parent. Offspring that are genetically identical to their parents are called clones.

Eukaryotic organisms often use sexual reproduction to generate offspring that contain a mixture of genetic material inherited from two different parents. The process of sexual reproduction alternates between forms that contain single copies of the genome (haploid) and double copies (diploid).[26] Haploid cells fuse and combine genetic material to create a diploid cell with paired chromosomes. Diploid organisms form haploids by dividing, without replicating their DNA, to create daughter cells that randomly inherit one of each pair of chromosomes. Most animals and many plants are diploid for most of their lifespan, with the haploid form reduced to single cell gametes such as sperm or eggs.

Although they do not use the haploid/diploid method of sexual reproduction, bacteria have many methods of acquiring new genetic information. Some bacteria can undergo conjugation, transferring a small circular piece of DNA to another bacterium.[40] Bacteria can also take up raw DNA fragments found in the environment and integrate them into their genomes, a phenomenon known as transformation.[41] These processes result in horizontal gene transfer, transmitting fragments of genetic information between organisms that would be otherwise unrelated.

Chromosomal Crossover and Genetic Linkage

Thomas Hunt Morgan's 1916 illustration of a double crossover between chromosomes

The diploid nature of chromosomes allows for genes on different chromosomes to assort independently during sexual reproduction, recombining to form new combinations of genes. Genes on the same chromosome would theoretically never recombine, however, were it not for the process of chromosomal crossover. During crossover, chromosomes exchange stretches of DNA, effectively shuffling the gene alleles between the chromosomes.[42] This process of chromosomal crossover generally occurs during meiosis, a series of cell divisions that creates haploid cells.

The probability of chromosomal crossover occurring between two given points on the chromosome is related to the distance between the points. For an arbitrarily long distance, the probability of crossover is high enough that the inheritance of the genes is effectively uncorrelated. For genes that are closer together, however, the lower probability of crossover means that the genes demonstrate genetic linkage-alleles for the two genes tend to be inherited together. The amounts of linkage between a series of genes can be combined to form a linear linkage map that roughly describes the arrangement of the genes along the chromosome.[43]

Genetic Code

Genes generally express their functional effect through the production of proteins, which are complex molecules responsible for most functions in the cell. Proteins are chains of amino acids, and the DNA sequence of a gene (through an RNA intermediate) is used to produce a specific protein sequence. This process begins with the production of an RNA molecule with a sequence matching the gene's DNA sequence, a process called transcription.

This messenger RNA molecule is then used to produce a corresponding amino acid sequence through a process called translation. Each group of three nucleotides in the sequence, called a codon, corresponds to one of the twenty possible amino acids in protein; this correspondence is called the genetic code.[44] The flow of information is unidirectional: information is transferred from nucleotide sequences into the amino acid sequence of proteins, but it never transfers from protein back into the sequence of DNA-a phenomenon Francis Crick called the central dogma of molecular biology.[45]

The specific sequence of amino acids results in a unique three-dimensional structure for that protein, and the three-dimensional structures of proteins are related to their functions.[46][47] Some are simple structural molecules, like the fibers formed by the protein collagen. Proteins can bind to other proteins and simple molecules, sometimes acting as enzymes by facilitating chemical reactions within the bound molecules (without changing the structure of the protein itself). Protein structure is dynamic; the protein hemoglobin bends into slightly different forms as it facilitates the capture, transport, and release of oxygen molecules within mammalian blood.

[54]

The dynamic structure of hemoglobin is responsible for its ability to transport oxygen within mammalian blood.

A single nucleotide difference within DNA can cause a change in the amino acid sequence of a protein. Because protein structures are the result of their amino acid sequences, some changes can dramatically change the properties of a protein by destabilizing the structure or changing the surface of the protein in a way that changes its interaction with other proteins and molecules. For example, sickle-cell anemia is a human genetic disease that results from a single base difference within the coding region for the β-globin section of hemoglobin, causing a single amino acid change that changes hemoglobin's physical properties.[48] Sickle-cell versions of hemoglobin stick to themselves, stacking to form fibers that distort the shape of red blood cells carrying the protein. These sickle-shaped cells no longer flow smoothly through blood vessels, having a tendency to clog or degrade, causing the medical problems associated with this disease.

Some genes are transcribed into RNA but are not translated into protein products-such RNA molecules are called non-coding RNA. In some cases, these products fold into structures which are involved in critical cell functions (e.g. ribosomal RNA and transfer RNA). RNA can also have regulatory effect through hybridization interactions with other RNA molecules (e.g. microRNA).

Nature versus Nurture

Although genes contain all the information an organism uses to function, the environment plays an important role in determining the ultimate phenotype-a phenomenon often referred to as "nature vs. nurture". The phenotype of an organism depends on the interaction of genetics with the environment. One example of this is the case of temperature-sensitive mutations. Often, a single amino acid change within the sequence of a protein does not change its behavior and interactions with other molecules, but it does destabilize the structure. In a high temperature environment, where molecules are moving more quickly and hitting each other, this results in the protein losing its structure and failing to function. In a low temperature environment, however, the protein's structure is stable and it functions normally. This type of mutation is visible in the coat coloration of Siamese cats, where a mutation in an enzyme responsible for pigment production causes it to destabilize and lose function at high temperatures.[49] The protein remains functional in areas of skin that are colder-legs, ears, tail, and face-and so the cat has dark fur at its extremities.

Environment also plays a dramatic role in effects of the human genetic disease phenylketonuria.[50] The mutation that causes phenylketonuria disrupts the ability of the body to break down the amino acid phenylalanine, causing a toxic build-up of an intermediate molecule that, in turn, causes severe symptoms of progressive mental retardation and seizures. If someone with the phenylketonuria mutation follows a strict diet that avoids this amino acid, however, they remain normal and healthy.

A popular method to determine how much role nature and nurture play is to study identical and fraternal twins or siblings of multiple birth. Because identical siblings come from the same zygote they are genetically the same. Fraternal siblings however are as different genetically from one another as normal siblings. By comparing how often the twin of a set has the same disorder between fraternal and identical twins, scientists can see whether there is more of a nature or nurture effect. One famous example of a multiple birth study includes the Genain quadruplets, who were identical quadruplets all diagnosed with schizophrenia.[51]

Regulation of Gene Expression

The genome of a given organism contains thousands of genes, but not all these genes need to be active at any given moment. A gene is expressed when it is being transcribed into mRNA (and translated into protein), and there exist many cellular methods of controlling the expression of genes such that proteins are produced only when needed by the cell. Transcription factors are regulatory proteins that bind to the start of genes, either promoting or inhibiting the transcription of the gene.[52] Within the genome of Escherichia coli bacteria, for example, there exists a series of genes necessary for the synthesis of the amino acid tryptophan. However, when tryptophan is already available to the cell, these genes for tryptophan synthesis are no longer needed. The presence of tryptophan directly affects the activity of the genes-tryptophan molecules bind to the tryptophan repressor (a transcription factor), changing the repressor's structure such that the repressor binds to the genes. The tryptophan repressor blocks the transcription and expression of the genes, thereby creating negative feedback regulation of the tryptophan synthesis process.[53]

Transcription factors bind to DNA, influencing the transcription of associated genes.

Differences in gene expression are especially clear within multi cellular organisms, where cells all contain the same genome but have very different structures and behaviors due to the expression of different sets of genes. All the cells in a multi cellular organism derive from a single cell, differentiating into variant cell types in response to external and intercellular signals and gradually establishing different patterns of gene expression to create different behaviors. As no single gene is responsible for the development of structures within multi cellular organisms, these patterns arise from the complex interactions between many cells.

Within eukaryotes there exist structural features of chromatin that influence the transcription of genes, often in the form of modifications to DNA and chromatin that are stably inherited by daughter cells.[54] These features are called "epigenetic" because they exist "on top" of the DNA sequence and retain inheritance from one cell generation to the next. Because of epigenetic features, different cell types grown within the same medium can retain very different properties. Although epigenetic features are generally dynamic over the course of development, some, like the phenomenon of paramutation, have multigenerational inheritance and exist as rare exceptions to the general rule of DNA as the basis for inheritance.[55]

Mutation

Gene duplication allows diversification by providing redundancy: one gene can mutate and lose its original function without harming the organism.

During the process of DNA replication, errors

occasionally occur in the polymerization of the second strand. These errors, called mutations, can have an impact on the phenotype of an organism, especially if they occur within the protein coding sequence of a gene. Error rates are usually very low-1 error in every 10-100 million bases-due to the "proofreading" ability of DNA polymerases.[56][57] (Without proofreading error rates are a thousand fold higher; because many viruses rely on DNA and RNA polymerases that lack proofreading ability, they experience higher mutation rates.) Processes that increase the rate of changes in DNA are called mutagenic: mutagenic chemicals promote errors in DNA replication, often by interfering with the structure of base-pairing, while UV radiation induces mutations by causing damage to the DNA structure.[58] Chemical damage to DNA occurs naturally as well, and cells use DNA repair mechanisms to repair mismatches and breaks in DNA-nevertheless, the repair sometimes fails to return the DNA to its original sequence.

In organisms that use chromosomal crossover to exchange DNA and recombine genes, errors in alignment during meiosis can also cause mutations.[59] Errors in crossover are especially likely when similar sequences cause partner chromosomes to adopt a mistaken alignment; this makes some regions in genomes more prone to mutating in this way. These errors create large structural changes in DNA sequence-duplications, inversions or deletions of entire regions, or the accidental exchanging of whole parts between different chromosomes (called translocation).

Evolution

Mutations alter an organism's genotype and occasionally this causes different phenotypes to appear. Most mutations have little effect on an organism's phenotype, health, or reproductive fitness. Mutations that do have an effect are usually deleterious, but occasionally some can be beneficial. Studies in the fly Drosophila melanogaster suggest that if a mutation changes a protein produced by a gene, about 70 percent of these mutations will be harmful with the remainder being either neutral or weakly beneficial.[60]

Population genetics studies the distribution of genetic differences within populations and how these distributions change over time.[61] Changes in the frequency of an allele in a population are mainly influenced by natural selection, where a given allele provides a selective or reproductive advantage to the organism,[62] as well as other factors such as genetic drift, artificial selection and migration.[63]

Over many generations, the genomes of organisms can change significantly, resulting in the phenomenon of evolution. Selection for beneficial mutations can cause a species to evolve into forms better able to survive in their environment, a process called adaptation.[64] New species are formed through the process of speciation, often caused by geographical separations that prevent populations from exchanging genes with each other.[65] The application of genetic principles to the study of population biology and evolution is referred to as the modern synthesis.

By comparing the homology between different species' genomes it is possible to calculate the evolutionary distance between them and when they may have diverged (called a molecular clock).[66] Genetic comparisons are generally considered a more accurate method of characterizing the relatedness between species than the comparison of phenotypic characteristics. The evolutionary distances between species can be used to form evolutionary trees; these trees represent the common descent and divergence of species over time, although they do not show the transfer of genetic material between unrelated species (known as horizontal gene transfer and most common in bacteria).

Although geneticists originally studied inheritance in a wide range of organisms, researchers began to specialize in studying the genetics of a particular subset of organisms. The fact that significant research already existed for a given organism would encourage new researchers to choose it for further study, and so eventually a few model organisms became the basis for most genetics research.[67] Common research topics in model organism genetics include the study of gene regulation and the involvement of genes in development and cancer.

Organisms were chosen, in part, for convenience-short generation times and easy genetic manipulation made some organisms popular genetics research tools. Widely used model organisms include the gut bacterium Escherichia coli, the plant Arabidopsis thaliana, baker's yeast (Saccharomyces cerevisiae), the nematode Caenorhabditis elegans, the common fruit fly (Drosophila melanogaster), and the common house mouse (Mus musculus).

Medical Genetics Research

Medical genetics seeks to understand how genetic variation relates to human health and disease.[68] When searching for an unknown gene that may be involved in a disease, researchers commonly use genetic linkage and genetic pedigree charts to find the location on the genome associated with the disease. At the population level, researchers take advantage of Mendelian randomization to look for locations in the genome that are associated with diseases, a technique especially useful for multigenic traits not clearly defined by a single gene.[69] Once a candidate gene is found, further research is often done on the corresponding gene (called an orthologous gene) in model organisms. In addition to studying genetic diseases, the increased availability of genotyping techniques has led to the field of pharmacogenetics-studying how genotype can affect drug responses.[70]

Individuals differ in their inherited tendency to develop cancer,[71] and cancer is a genetic disease.[72] The process of cancer development in the body is a combination of events. Mutations occasionally occur within cells in the body as they divide. Although these mutations will not be inherited by any offspring, they can affect the behavior of cells, sometimes causing them to grow and divide more frequently. There are biological mechanisms that attempt to stop this process; signals are given to inappropriately dividing cells that should trigger cell death, but sometimes additional mutations occur that cause cells to ignore these messages. An internal process of natural selection occurs within the body and eventually mutations accumulate within cells to promote their own growth, creating a cancerous tumor that grows and invades various tissues of the body.

Research Techniques

DNA can be manipulated in the laboratory. Restriction enzymes are commonly used enzymes that cut DNA at specific sequences, producing predictable fragments of DNA.[73] DNA fragments can be visualized through use of gel electrophoresis, which separates fragments according to their length.

The use of ligation enzymes allows DNA fragments to be connected, and by ligating fragments of DNA together from different sources, researchers can create recombinant DNA. Often associated with genetically modified organisms, recombinant DNA is commonly used in the context of plasmids-short circular DNA fragments with a few genes on them. By inserting plasmids into bacteria and growing those bacteria on plates of agar (to isolate clones of bacteria cells), researchers can clonally amplify the inserted fragment of DNA (a process known as molecular cloning). (Cloning can also refer to the creation of clonal organisms, through various techniques.)

DNA can also be amplified using a procedure called the polymerase chain reaction (PCR).[74] By using specific short sequences of DNA, PCR can isolate and exponentially amplify a targeted region of DNA. Because it can amplify from extremely small amounts of DNA, PCR is also often used to detect the presence of specific DNA sequences.

DNA Sequencing and Genomics

One of the most fundamental technologies developed to study genetics, DNA sequencing allows researchers to determine the sequence of nucleotides in DNA fragments. Developed in 1977 by Frederick Sanger and coworkers, chain-termination sequencing is now routinely used to sequence DNA fragments.[75] With this technology, researchers have been able to study the molecular sequences associated with many human diseases.

As sequencing has become less expensive, researchers have sequenced the genomes of many organisms, using computational tools to stitch together the sequences of many different fragments (a process called genome assembly).[76] These technologies were used to sequence the human genome, leading to the completion of the Human Genome Project in 2003.[23] New high-throughput sequencing technologies are dramatically lowering the cost of DNA sequencing, with many researchers hoping to bring the cost of resequencing a human genome down to a thousand dollars.[77]

The large amount of sequence data available has created the field of genomics, research that uses computational tools to search for and analyze patterns in the full genomes of organisms. Genomics can also be considered a subfield of bioinformatics, which uses computational approaches to analyze large sets of biological data.

Notes

1. Genetikos, Henry George Liddell, Robert Scott, "A Greek-English Lexicon", at Perseus

2. Genesis, Henry George Liddell, Robert Scott, "A Greek-English Lexicon", at Perseus

3. Online Etymology Dictionary

4. Griffiths, William M.; Miller, Jeffrey H.; Suzuki, David T. et al., eds (2000)."Genetics and the Organism: Introduction". An Introduction to Genetic Analysis (7th ed.). New York: W. H. Freeman. ISBN 0-7167-3520-2.

5. Hartl D, Jones E (2005)

6. Weiling, F (1991). "Historical study: Johann Gregor Mendel 1822-1884.".American journal of medical genetics 40 (1): 1-25; discussion 26.doi:10.1002/ajmg.1320400103. PMID 1887835.

7. Lamarck, J-B (2008). In Encyclopædia Britannica. Retrieved fromEncyclopædia Britannica Online on 16 March 2008.

8. Peter J. Bowler, The Mendelian Revolution: The Emergency of Hereditarian Concepts in Modern Science and

Society (Baltimore: Johns Hopkins University Press, 1989): chapters 2 & 3.

9. a b Blumberg, Roger B.. "Mendel's Paper in English".

10. genetics, n., Oxford English Dictionary, 3rd ed.

11. Bateson W. "Letter from William Bateson to Alan Sedgwick in 1905". The John Innes Centre. Retrieved 15 March 2008.. Note that the letter was to an Adam Sedgwick, a zoologist at Trinity College, Cambridge, not "Alan", and not to be confused with the renowned British geologist, Adam Sedgwick, who lived some time earlier.

12. genetic, adj., Oxford English Dictionary, 3rd ed.

13. Bateson, W (1907). "The Progress of Genetic Research". In Wilks, W.Report of the Third 1906 International Conference on Genetics: Hybridization (the cross-breeding of genera or species), the cross-breeding of varieties, and general plant breeding. London: Royal Horticultural Society.

Initially titled the "International Conference on Hybridisation and Plant Breeding", Wilks changed the title for publication as a result of Bateson's speech.[citation needed]

14. Moore, John A. (1983). "Thomas Hunt Morgan-The Geneticist". Integrative and Comparative Biology 23: 855.

doi:10.1093/icb/23.4.855.

15. Sturtevant AH (1913). "The linear arrangement of six sex-linked factors in Drosophila, as shown by their mode of association". Journal of Experimental Biology 14: 43-59.

16. Avery, OT; MacLeod, CM; McCarty, M (1944). "STUDIES ON THE CHEMICAL NATURE OF THE SUBSTANCE INDUCING TRANSFORMATION OF PNEUMOCOCCAL TYPES : INDUCTION OF TRANSFORMATION BY A DESOXYRIBONUCLEIC ACID FRACTION ISOLATED FROM PNEUMOCOCCUS TYPE III.". The Journal of experimental medicine 79 (2): 137-58. doi:10.1084/jem.79.2.137. PMID 19871359. Reprint: Avery, OT; Macleod, CM; Mccarty, M (1979). "Studies on the chemical nature of the substance inducing transformation of pneumococcal types. Inductions of transformation by a desoxyribonucleic acid fraction isolated from pneumococcus type III.". The Journal of experimental medicine 149 (2): 297-326. doi:10.1084/jem.149.2.297. PMID 33226.

17. Hershey, AD; Chase, M (1952). "Independent functions of viral protein and nucleic acid in growth of bacteriophage". The Journal of general physiology 36 (1): 39-56. doi:10.1085/jgp.36.1.39. PMID 12981234.

18. Judson, Horace (1979). The Eighth Day of Creation:

Makers of the Revolution in Biology. Cold Spring Harbor Laboratory Press. pp. 51-169.ISBN 0-87969-477-7.

19. Watson, J. D.; Crick, FH (1953). "Molecular Structure of Nucleic Acids: A Structure for Deoxyribose Nucleic Acid". Nature 171 (4356): 737.doi:10.1038/171737a0. PMID 13054692.

20. Watson, J. D.; Crick, FH (1953). "Genetical Implications of the Structure of Deoxyribonucleic Acid". Nature 171 (4361): 964. doi:10.1038/171964b0.PMID 13063483.

21. Sanger, F; Nicklen, S; Coulson, AR (1977). "DNA sequencing with chain-terminating inhibitors". Proceedings of the National Academy of Sciences of the United States of America 74 (12): 5463-7.doi:10.1073/pnas.74.12.5463. PMID 271968.

22. Saiki, RK; Scharf, S; Faloona, F; Mullis, KB; Horn, GT; Erlich, HA; Arnheim, N (1985). "Enzymatic amplification of beta-globin genomic sequences and restriction site analysis for diagnosis of sickle cell anemia.". Science 230(4732): 1350-4. doi:10.1126/science.2999980. PMID 2999980.

23. a b "Human Genome Project Information". Human Genome Project. Retrieved 15 March 2008.

24.	Griffiths, William M.; Miller, Jeffrey H.; Suzuki, David T. et al., eds (2000)."Patterns of Inheritance: Introduction". An Introduction to Genetic Analysis(7th ed.). New York: W. H. Freeman. ISBN 0-7167-3520-2.

25.	Griffiths, William M.; Miller, Jeffrey H.; Suzuki, David T. et al., eds (2000)."Mendel's experiments". An Introduction to Genetic Analysis (7th ed.). New York: W. H. Freeman. ISBN 0-7167-3520-2.

26.	a b c Griffiths, William M.; Miller, Jeffrey H.; Suzuki, David T. et al., eds (2000)."Mendelian genetics in eukaryotic life cycles". An Introduction to Genetic Analysis (7th ed.). New York: W. H. Freeman. ISBN 0-7167-3520-2.

27.	Griffiths, William M.; Miller, Jeffrey H.; Suzuki, David T. et al., eds (2000)."Interactions between the alleles of one gene". An Introduction to Genetic Analysis (7th ed.). New York: W. H. Freeman. ISBN 0-7167-3520-2.

28.	Cheney, Richard W.. "Genetic Notation". Retrieved 18 March 2008.

29.	Griffiths, William M.; Miller, Jeffrey H.; Suzuki, David T. et al., eds (2000)."Human Genetics". An Introduction to Genetic Analysis (7th ed.). New York: W. H. Freeman. ISBN 0-7167-3520-2.

30.	Griffiths, William M.; Miller, Jeffrey H.; Suzuki,

David T. et al., eds (2000)."Gene interaction and modified dihybrid ratios". An Introduction to Genetic Analysis (7th ed.). New York: W. H. Freeman. ISBN 0-7167-3520-2.

31.   Mayeux, R (2005). "Mapping the new frontier: complex genetic disorders.".The Journal of clinical investigation 115 (6): 1404-7.doi:10.1172/JCI25421. PMID 15931374.

32.   Griffiths, William M.; Miller, Jeffrey H.; Suzuki, David T. et al., eds (2000)."Quantifying heritability". An Introduction to Genetic Analysis (7th ed.). New York: W. H. Freeman. ISBN 0-7167-3520-2.

33.   Luke, A; Guo, X; Adeyemo, AA; Wilks, R; Forrester, T; Lowe W, W; Comuzzie, AG; Martin, LJ et al. (2001). "Heritability of obesity-related traits among Nigerians, Jamaicans and US black people.". International journal of obesity and related metabolic disorders 25 (7): 1034-41.doi:10.1038/sj.ijo.0801650. PMID 11443503.

34.   Pearson, H (2006). "Genetics: what is a gene?". Nature 441 (7092): 398-401. doi:10.1038/441398a. PMID 16724031.

35.   Prescott, L (1993). Microbiology. Wm. C. Brown Publishers.ISBN 0697013723.

36.   Griffiths, William M.; Miller, Jeffrey H.; Suzuki,

David T. et al., eds (2000)."Mechanism of DNA Replication". An Introduction to Genetic Analysis (7th ed.). New York: W. H. Freeman. ISBN 0-7167-3520-2.

37. Gregory, SG; Barlow, KF; Mclay, KE; Kaul, R; Swarbreck, D; Dunham, A; Scott, CE; Howe, KL et al. (2006). "The DNA sequence and biological annotation of human chromosome 1.". Nature 441 (7091): 315-21.doi:10.1038/nature04727. PMID 16710414.

38. Alberts et al. (2002), II.4. DNA and chromosomes: Chromosomal DNA and Its Packaging in the Chromatin Fiber

39. Griffiths, William M.; Miller, Jeffrey H.; Suzuki, David T. et al., eds (2000). "Sex chromosomes and sex-linked inheritance". An Introduction to Genetic Analysis (7th ed.). New York: W. H. Freeman. ISBN 0-7167-3520-2.

40. Griffiths, William M.; Miller, Jeffrey H.; Suzuki, David T. et al., eds (2000)."Bacterial conjugation". An Introduction to Genetic Analysis (7th ed.). New York: W. H. Freeman. ISBN 0-7167-3520-2.

41. Griffiths, William M.; Miller, Jeffrey H.; Suzuki, David T. et al., eds (2000)."Bacterial transformation". An Introduction to Genetic Analysis (7th ed.). New York: W. H. Freeman. ISBN 0-7167-3520-2.

42. Griffiths, William M.; Miller, Jeffrey H.; Suzuki, David T. et al., eds (2000)."Nature of crossing-over". An Introduction to Genetic Analysis (7th ed.). New York: W. H. Freeman. ISBN 0-7167-3520-2.

43. Griffiths, William M.; Miller, Jeffrey H.; Suzuki, David T. et al., eds (2000)."Linkage maps". An Introduction to Genetic Analysis (7th ed.). New York: W. H. Freeman. ISBN 0-7167-3520-2.

44. Berg JM, Tymoczko JL, Stryer L, Clarke ND (2002). "I. 5. DNA, RNA, and the Flow of Genetic Information: Amino Acids Are Encoded by Groups of Three Bases Starting from a Fixed Point". Biochemistry (5th ed.). New York: W. H. Freeman and Company.

45. Crick, F (1970). "Central dogma of molecular biology.". Nature 227(5258): 561-3. doi:10.1038/227561a0. PMID 4913914.

46. Alberts et al. (2002), I.3. Proteins: The Shape and Structure of Proteins

47. Alberts et al. (2002), I.3. Proteins: Protein Function

48. "How Does Sickle Cell Cause Disease?". Brigham and Women's Hospital: Information Center for Sickle Cell and Thalassemic Disorders. 11 April 2002. Retrieved 23 July 2007.

49. Imes, DL; Geary, LA; Grahn, RA; Lyons, LA (2006). "Albinism in the domestic cat (Felis catus) is associated with a tyrosinase (TYR) mutation.".Animal genetics 37 (2): 175-8. doi:10.1111/j.1365-2052.2005.01409.x.PMID 16573534.

50. "MedlinePlus: Phenylketonuria". NIH: National Library of Medicine. Retrieved 15 March 2008.

51. Rosenthal, David (1964). The Genain quadruplets; a case study and theoretical analysis of heredity and environment in schizophrenia.. New York: Basic Books. ISBN B0000CM68F.

52. Brivanlou, AH; Darnell Je, JE (2002). "Signal transduction and the control of gene expression.". Science 295 (5556): 813-8.doi:10.1126/science.1066355. PMID 11823631.

53. Alberts et al. (2002), II.3. Control of Gene Expression - The Tryptophan Repressor Is a Simple Switch That Turns Genes On and Off in Bacteria

54. Jaenisch, R; Bird, A (2003). "Epigenetic regulation of gene expression: how the genome integrates intrinsic and environmental signals.". Nature genetics33 Suppl: 245-54. doi:10.1038/ng1089. PMID 12610534.

55. Chandler, VL (2007). "Paramutation: from maize to mice.". Cell 128 (4): 641-5. doi:10.1016/j.cell.2007.02.007.

PMID 17320501.

56. Griffiths, William M.; Miller, Jeffrey H.; Suzuki, David T. et al., eds (2000)."Spontaneous mutations". An Introduction to Genetic Analysis (7th ed.). New York: W. H. Freeman. ISBN 0-7167-3520-2.

57. Freisinger, E; Grollman, AP; Miller, H; Kisker, C (2004). "Lesion (in)tolerance reveals insights into DNA replication fidelity.". The EMBO journal 23 (7): 1494-505. doi:10.1038/sj.emboj.7600158.PMID 15057282.

58. Griffiths, William M.; Miller, Jeffrey H.; Suzuki, David T. et al., eds (2000)."Induced mutations". An Introduction to Genetic Analysis (7th ed.). New York: W. H. Freeman. ISBN 0-7167-3520-2.

59. Griffiths, William M.; Miller, Jeffrey H.; Suzuki, David T. et al., eds (2000)."Chromosome Mutation I: Changes in Chromosome Structure: Introduction". An Introduction to Genetic Analysis (7th ed.). New York: W. H. Freeman. ISBN 0-7167-3520-2.

60. Sawyer, SA; Parsch, J; Zhang, Z; Hartl, DL (2007). "Prevalence of positive selection among nearly neutral amino acid replacements in Drosophila.".Proceedings of the National Academy of Sciences of the United States of America 104 (16): 6504-10.

doi:10.1073/pnas.0701572104.PMID 17409186.

61. Griffiths, William M.; Miller, Jeffrey H.; Suzuki, David T. et al., eds (2000)."Variation and its modulation". An Introduction to Genetic Analysis (7th ed.). New York: W. H. Freeman. ISBN 0-7167-3520-2.

62. Griffiths, William M.; Miller, Jeffrey H.; Suzuki, David T. et al., eds (2000)."Selection". An Introduction to Genetic Analysis (7th ed.). New York: W. H. Freeman. ISBN 0-7167-3520-2.

63. Griffiths, William M.; Miller, Jeffrey H.; Suzuki, David T. et al., eds (2000)."Random events". An Introduction to Genetic Analysis (7th ed.). New York: W. H. Freeman. ISBN 0-7167-3520-2.

64. Darwin, Charles (1859). On the Origin of Species (1st ed.). London: John Murray. pp. 1. ISBN 0801413192.. Related earlier ideas were acknowledged in Darwin, Charles (1861). On the Origin of Species (3rd ed.). London: John Murray. xiii. ISBN 0801413192.

65. Gavrilets, S (2003). "Perspective: models of speciation: what have we learned in 40 years?". Evolution; international journal of organic evolution 57(10): 2197-215. doi:10.1554/02-727. PMID 14628909.

66. Wolf, YI; Rogozin, IB; Grishin, NV; Koonin, EV

(2002). "Genome trees and the tree of life.". Trends in genetics 18 (9): 472-9. doi:10.1016/S0168-9525(02)02744-0. PMID 12175808.

67.   "The Use of Model Organisms in Instruction". University of Wisconsin: Wisconsin Outreach Research Modules. Retrieved 15 March 2008.

68.   "NCBI: Genes and Disease". NIH: National Center for Biotechnology Information. Retrieved 15 March 2008.

69.   Davey Smith, G; Ebrahim, S (2003). "'Mendelian randomization': can genetic epidemiology contribute to understanding environmental determinants of disease?". International journal of epidemiology 32 (1): 1-22.doi:10.1093/ije/dyg070. PMID 12689998.

70.   "Pharmacogenetics Fact Sheet". NIH: National Institute of General Medical Sciences. Retrieved 15 March 2008.

71.   Frank, SA (2004). "Genetic predisposition to cancer - insights from population genetics". Nature reviews. Genetics 5 (10): 764-72.doi:10.1038/nrg1450. PMID 15510167.

72.   Strachan T, Read AP (1999). Human Molecular Genetics 2 (second ed.). John Wiley & Sons Inc..Chapter 18: Cancer Genetics

73.   Lodish et al. (2000), Chapter 7: 7.1. DNA Cloning with Plasmid Vectors

74.   Lodish et al. (2000), Chapter 7: 7.7. Polymerase Chain Reaction: An Alternative to Cloning

75.   Brown TA (2002). "Section 2, Chapter 6: 6.1. The Methodology for DNA Sequencing". Genomes 2 (2nd ed.). Oxford: Bios. ISBN 1 85996 228 9.

76.   Brown (2002), Section 2, Chapter 6: 6.2. Assembly of a Contiguous DNA Sequence

77.   Service, RF (2006). "Gene sequencing. The race for the $1000 genome.".Science 311 (5767): 1544-6. doi:10.1126/science.311.5767.1544.PMID 16543431.

References

Alberts B, Johnson A, Lewis J, Raff M, Roberts K, and Walter P (2002).Molecular Biology of the Cell (4th ed.). New York: Garland Science. ISBN 0-8153-3218-1.

Griffiths, William M.; Miller, Jeffrey H.; Suzuki, David T. et al., eds (2000).An Introduction to Genetic Analysis (7th ed.). New York: W. H. Freeman.ISBN 0-7167-3520-2.

Hartl D, Jones E (2005). Genetics: Analysis of Genes and Genomes (6th ed.). Jones & Bartlett. ISBN 0-7637-1511-5.

Lodish H, Berk A, Zipursky LS, Matsudaira P, Baltimore D, and Darnell J (2000). Molecular Cell Biology (4th ed.). New

York: Scientific American Books. ISBN 0-7167-3136-3.

Wikipedia. Genetics. Article Retrieved October 10th, 2010 from: <http://en.wikipedia.org/wiki/Genetics>.

Glossary of Medical Terms

Abnormal: Not normal. Deviating from the usual position, condition, structure or behavior. An abnormal growth could indicate a premalignant or malignant condition. In other words, an abnormal growth could indicate cancer

Acquired: An acquired condition is one that isn't present at birth. In other words, it is a condition that is not inherited.

Acute: A condition with an abrupt onset. A brain aneurism is said to be acute if it comes on suddenly. An acute condition could also describe an illness of short duration that rapidly progresses and requires urgent care.

Airway: The trachea. A method of preventing sensation, used to eliminate pain. The loss or prevention of pain, as caused by anesthesia.

Aneurysm or Aneurism: An abnormal blood-filled swelling of an artery or vein, resulting from a localized weakness in the wall of the vessel.

Angiography: A medical imaging technique in which an X-ray image is taken to visualize the inside of blood vessels and organs of the body, with particular interest in the arteries, veins and the heart chambers.

Artery: An efferent blood vessel from the heart, conveying blood away from the heart regardless of oxygenation status.

Autopsy: A dissection performed on a cadaver to find possible cause(s) of death. An after-the-fact examination, especially of the causes of a failure.

Berry aneurysm: An aneurism that looks like a berry. It usually happens where a cerebral artery leaves the circular artery at the base of the brain.

Blood pressure: The pressure exerted by the blood against the walls of the arteries and veins; it varies during the heartbeat cycle, and according to a person's age, health and physical condition. The great majority of people who have serious conditions from high blood pressure suffer debilitating illness.

Brain: The control center of the central nervous system of an animal located in the skull which is responsible for perception, cognition, attention, memory, emotion, and action.

Brain aneurysm: See berry aneurysm.

Brain swelling: See: Cerebral edema.

Breathing: The act of respiration; a single instance of this.

Calcium: A mineral stored in the bones. Calcium is added to bones by osteoblasts and is removed osteoclasts. This mineral s essential for healthy bones and regulates muscle contraction, heart action, nervous system maintenance, and normal blood clotting. Food sources of calcium include dairy foods, some leafy green vegetables such as broccoli and collards, canned salmon, clams, oysters, calcium-fortified foods, and tofu.

Calcium channel blocker: A drug that blocks calcium from entering the heart and artery muscle, preventing narrowing of the arteries.

Cardiovascular: Relating to the circulatory system, that is the heart and blood vessels.

Catheter: small tube inserted into a body cavity to remove fluid, create an opening, distend a passageway or administer a drug

Cell: The basic unit of a living organism, surrounded by a cell membrane.

Cerebral: Of, or relating to the brain or cerebral cortex of the brain.

Cerebral aneurysm: See: Berry aneurysm.

Cholesterol: A sterollipid synthesized by the liver and transported in the bloodstream to the membranes of all animal cells; it plays a central role in many biochemical processes and, as a lipoprotein that coats the walls of blood vessels, is associated with cardiovascular disease.

Circle of Willis: An arterial circle at the base of the brain. Circulation: The movement of the blood in the blood-vascular system, by which it is brought into close relations with almost every living elementary constituent.

Cocaine: A stimulant narcotic in the form of a white powder that users generally self-administer by insufflation through the nose. Any derivative of cocaine. Extracted from the leaves of the coca scrub (Erythroxylon coca) indigenous to the Andean highlands of South America.

Coma: A state of sleep from which one may not wake up, usually induced by some form of trauma.

Compression (medicine): Pressing together. As in a compression fracture, nerve compression , or spinal cord compression.

Compression (embryology): To shorten in time.

Connective tissue: type of tissue found in animals whose main function is binding other tissue systems (such as muscle to skin) or organs and consists of the following three elements: cells, fibers and a ground substance (or extracellular matrix).

Contrast: Any substance, such as barium sulfate, used in radiography to increase the visibility of internal structures

CT scan: Computerized tomography scan. Pictures of the body created by a computer where multiple X-ray images are turned into pictures on a screen.

Cysts: A pouch or sac without opening, usually membranous and containing morbid matter, which develops in one of the natural cavities or in the substance of an organ.

Dizziness: he state of being dizzy; the sensation of instability.

Doppler ultrasound: A type of ultrasound that detects and measures blood flow.

Ehlers-Danlos syndrome: A heritable disorder of connective tissue with easy bruising, joint hypermobility (loose joints), skin laxity, and weakness of tissues.

Emergency department: The department of a hospital that treats emergencies.

Extended family: a family consisting of parents and children, along with either grandparents, grandchildren, aunts or uncles etc.

Extremity: the most extreme or furthest point of something.

1.   An extreme measure.

2.   A hand or foot.

Genetic: (genetics) relating to genetics or genes. Caused by genes.

Groin: The long narrow depression of the human body that separates the trunk from the legs.

Headache: A pain or ache in the head.

Hemorrhage: A heavy release of blood within or from the body.

High blood pressure: Hypertension: a repeatedly elevated blood pressure exceeding 140 over 90 mmHg -- a systolic pressure above 140 with a diastolic pressure above 90.

Inheritance: The hereditary passing of biological attributes from ancestors to their offspring.

Interventional: Intervening, interfering or interceding with the intent of modifying the outcome. For example, an interventional radiologist.

Intracranial: f or pertaining to the brain or inside of the head. Within the cranium.

Kidney: an organ in the body that produces urine.

Lifetime risk: The risk of developing a particular disease or dying from that disease during your lifetime.

Long-term memory: Permanent storage, management, and retrieval of information for later use.

Lumbar: Related to the lower back or loin.

Lumbar puncture: A diagnostic and at times therapeutic procedure performed to collect a sample of cerebrospinal fluid for biochemical, microbiological, and cytological analysis, or rarely to relieve increased intracranial pressure.

Marfan syndrome: A genetic disorder of the connective tissue that causes defects in the heart valves and aorta. Characterized by abnormalities of the eyes, skeleton, and cardiovascular system.

Memory: 1. The ability to recover information about past events or knowledge. 2. The process of recovering information about past events or knowledge. 3. Cognitive reconstruction. The brain engages in a remarkable reshuffling process in an attempt to extract what is general and what is particular about each passing moment.

Migraine: Usually, periodic attacks of headaches on one or both sides of the head. These may be accompanied by nausea, vomiting, increased sensitivity of the eyes to light (photophobia), increased sensitivity to sound (phonophobia), dizziness, blurred vision, cognitive disturbances, and other symptoms. Some migraines do not include headache, and migraines may or may not be preceded by an aura.

MRI: Abbreviation and nickname for magnetic resonance imaging. For more information, see: Magnetic Resonance Imaging; Paul C. Lauterbur ; Peter Mansfield .

Nausea: Nausea, is the urge to vomit. It can be brought by many causes including, systemic illnesses, such as influenza, medications, pain, and inner ear disease. When nausea and/or vomiting are persistent, or when they are accompanied by other severe symptoms such as abdominal pain, jaundice , fever, or bleeding, a physician should be consulted.

Neck: The part of the body joining the head to the shoulders. Also, any narrow or constricted part of a bone or organ that joins its parts as, for example, the neck of the femur bone.

Nerve: A bundle of fibers that uses chemical and electrical signals to transmit sensory and motor information from one body part to another. See: Nervous system.

Nerve cell: See: Neuron.

Neurofibromatosis: A genetic disorder of the nervous system that primarily affects the development and growth of neural (nerve) cell tissues, causes tumors to grow on nerves, and may produce other abnormalities.

Neurological: Having to do with the nerves or the nervous system.

Neurology: The medical specialty concerned with the diagnosis and treatment of disorders of the nervous system -- the brain, the spinal cord, and the nerves.

Neuroradiology: The field within radiology that specializes in the use of radioactive substances, x-rays and scanning devices for the diagnosis and treatment of diseases of the nervous system. Neuroradiology involves the clinical imaging, therapy, and basic science of the central and peripheral nervous system , including but not limited to the brain, spine , head and neck , interventional procedures, techniques in imaging and intervention , and related educational, socioeconomic, and medicolegal issues.

Neurosurgeon: A physician trained in surgery of the nervous system and who specializes in surgery on the brain and other parts of the nervous system. Sometimes called a "brain surgeon."

NIH: The National Institutes of Health. The NIH is an important U.S. health agency. It is devoted to medical research. Administratively under the Department of Health and Human Services (HHS), the NIH consists of 20-some separate Institutes and Centers. NIH's program activities are represented by these Institutes and Centers.

Onset: In medicine, the first appearance of the signs or symptoms of an illness as, for example, the onset of rheumatoid arthritis. There is always an onset to a disease but never to the return to good health. The default setting is good health.

Outpatient: A patient who is not an inpatient (not hospitalized) but instead is cared for elsewhere -- as in a doctor's office, clinic, or day surgery center. The term outpatient dates back at least to 1715. Outpatient care today is also called ambulatory care.

Pain: An unpleasant sensation that can range from mild, localized discomfort to agony. Pain has both physical and emotional components. The physical part of pain results from nerve stimulation. Pain may be contained to a discrete area, as in an injury, or it can be more diffuse, as in disorders like fibromyalgia. Pain is mediated by specific nerve fibers that carry the pain impulses to the brain where their conscious appreciation may be modified by many factors.

Pharmacy: A location where prescription drugs are sold. A pharmacy is, by law, constantly supervised by a licensed pharmacist.

Polycystic kidney disease: One of the genetic disorders characterized by the development of innumerable cysts in the kidneys. These cysts are filled with fluid, and replace much of the mass of the kidneys. This reduces kidney function, leading to kidney failure.

Pupil: The opening of the iris. The pupil may appear to open (dilate) and close (constrict) but it is really the iris that is the prime mover; the pupil is merely the absence of iris. The pupil determines how much light is let into the eye. Both pupils are usually of equal size. If they are not, that is termed anisocoria (from "a-", not + "iso", equal + "kore", pupil = not equal pupils).

Radiologic: Having to do with radiology.

Radiologist: A physician specialized in radiology, the branch of medicine that uses ionizing and nonionizing radiation for the diagnosis and treatment of disease.

Residual: Something left behind. With residual disease, the disease has not been eradicated.

Risk factor: Something that increases a person's chances of developing a disease.

Rupture: A break or tear in any organ (such as the spleen) or soft tissue (such as the achilles tendon). Rupture of the appendix is more likely among uninsured and minority children when they develop appendicitis.

Saccular: From the Latin "sacculus" meaning a small pouch. As for example the alveolar saccules (little air pouches) within the lungs.

Saccular aneurysm: An aneurysm that resembles a small sack. A berry aneurysm is typically saccular. An aneurysm is a localized widening (dilatation) of an artery, vein, or the heart. At the area of an aneurysm, there is typically a bulge and the wall is weakened and may rupture. The word "aneurysm" comes from the Greek "aneurysma" meaning "a widening."

Scan: As a noun, the data or image obtained from the examination of organs or regions of the body by gathering information with a sensing device.

Seizure: Uncontrolled electrical activity in the brain, which may produce a physical convulsion, minor physical signs, thought disturbances, or a combination of symptoms.

Sensitivity: 1. In psychology, the quality of being sensitive. As, for example, sensitivity training, training in small groups to develop a sensitive awareness and understanding of oneself and of ones relationships with others. 2. In disease epidemiology, the ability of a system to detect epidemics and other changes in disease occurrence. 3. In screening for a disease, the proportion of persons with the disease who are correctly identified by a screening test. 4. In the definition of a disease, the proportion of persons with the disease who are correctly identified by defined criteria.

Skull: The skull is a collection of bones which encase the brain and give form to the head and face. The bones of the skull include the following: the frontal, parietal, occipital, temporal, sphenoid, ethmoid, zygomatic, maxilla, nasal, vomer, palatine, inferior concha, and mandible.

Spasm: A brief, automatic jerking movement. A muscle spasm can be quite painful, with the muscle clenching tightly. A spasm of the coronary artery can cause angina. Spasms in various types of tissue may be caused by stress, medication, over-exercise, or other factors.

Spinal cord: The major column of nerve tissue that is connected to the brain and lies within the vertebral canal and from which the spinal nerves emerge. Thirty-one pairs of spinal nerves originate in the spinal cord: 8 cervical, 12 thoracic , 5 lumbar, 5 sacral, and 1 coccygeal. The spinal cord and the brain constitute the central nervous system (CNS). The spinal cord consists of nerve fibers that transmit impulses to and from the brain. Like the brain, the spinal cord is covered by three connective-tissue envelopes called the meninges . The space between the outer and middle envelopes is filled with cerebrospinal fluid (CSF), a clear colorless fluid that cushions the spinal cord against jarring shock. Also known simply as the cord.

Spinal tap: Also known as a lumbar puncture or "LP", a spinal tap is a procedure whereby spinal fluid is removed from the spinal canal for the purpose of diagnostic testing. It is particularly helpful in the diagnosis of inflammatory diseases of the central nervous system, especially infections, such as meningitis. It can also provide clues to the diagnosis of stroke, spinal cord tumor and cancer in the central nervous system.

Stress: Forces from the outside world impinging on the individual. Stress is a normal part of life that can help us learn and grow. Conversely, stress can cause us significant problems.

Stroke: The sudden death of some brain cells due to a lack of oxygen when the blood flow to the brain is impaired by blockage or rupture of an artery to the brain. A stroke is also called a cerebrovascular accident or, for short, a CVA.

Subarachnoid: Literally, beneath the arachnoid, the middle of three membranes that cover the central nervous system. In practice, subarachnoid usually refers to the space between the arachnoid and the pia mater, the innermost membrane surrounding the central nervous system.

Subarachnoid hemorrhage: Bleeding within the head into the space between two membranes that surround the brain. The bleeding is beneath the arachnoid membrane and just above the pia mater. (The arachnoid is the middle of three membranes around the brain while the pia mater is the innermost one.)

Surgery: The word "surgery" has multiple meanings. It is the branch of medicine concerned with diseases and conditions which require or are amenable to operative procedures. Surgery is the work done by a surgeon. By analogy, the work of an editor wielding his pen as a scalpel is s form of surgery. A surgery in England (and some other countries) is a physician's or dentist's office.

Swelling of the brain: See: Cerebral edema.

Symptom: Any subjective evidence of disease. Anxiety, lower back pain, and fatigue are all symptoms. They are sensations only the patient can perceive. In contrast, a sign is objective evidence of disease. A bloody nose is a sign. It is evident to the patient, doctor, nurse and other observers.

Syndrome: A set of signs and symptoms that tend to occur together and which reflect the presence of a particular disease or an increased chance of developing a particular disease.

Temple: An area just behind and to the side of the forehead and the eye, above the side of the check bone (the zygomatic arch) and in front of the ear.

Tension: 1) The pressure within a vessel, such as blood pressure: the pressure within the blood vessels. For example, elevated blood pressure is referred to as hypertension. 2) Stress, especially stress that is translated into clenched scalp muscles and bottled-up emotions or anxiety. This is the type of tension blamed for tension headaches.

Therapeutic: Relating to therapeutics, that part of medicine concerned specifically with the treatment of disease. The therapeutic dose of a drug is the amount needed to treat a disease.

Throat: The throat is the anterior (front) portion of the neck beginning at the back of the mouth , consisting anatomically of the pharynx and larynx . The throat contains the trachea and a portion of the esophagus.

Tobacco: A South American herb, formally known as Nicotiana tabacum, whose leaves contain 2-8% nicotine and serve as the source of smoking and smokeless tobacco.

Transcranial: Through the cranium. As, for example, in transcranial magnetic stimulation.

Ultrasound : High-frequency sound waves. Ultrasound waves can be bounced off of tissues using special devices. The echoes are then converted into a picture called a sonogram. Ultrasound imaging, referred to as ultrasonography, allows physicians and patients to get an inside view of soft tissues and body cavities, without using invasive techniques. Ultrasound is often used to examine a fetus during pregnancy There is no convincing evidence for any danger from ultrasound during pregnancy.

Vessel: A tube in the body that carries fluids: blood vessels or lymph vessels.

Visual field: The entire area that can be seen when the eye is directed forward, including that which is seen with peripheral vision.

X-ray: 1. High-energy radiation with waves shorter than those of visible light. X-rays possess the properties of penetrating most substances (to varying extents), of acting on a photographic film or plate (permitting radiography), and of causing a fluorescent screen to give off light (permitting fluoroscopy). In low doses X-rays are used for making images that help to diagnose disease, and in high doses to treat cancer. Formerly called a Roentgen ray. 2. An image obtained by means of X-rays.

Appendix A: Internet Resources / Further Reading

The following Internet resources may be helpful in answering any health or medical questions you may have. The sites were chosen because of their superior content, accuracy, and authority.

Print Publications Online

American Family Physician

<http://www.aafp.org/online/en/home/publications/journals/afp.html>

A full-text, online version of the esteemed journal. Contains excellent review articles on clinical medicine. Many come with patient education information.

Merck Manual of Diagnosis and Therapy, 17th ed.

<http://www.merck.com/mmpe/index.html>

A medical guide for professionals, available online. Contains technical information for a host of diseases along with their corresponding diagnosis and treatment suggestions.

Merck Manual of Geriatrics

<http://www.merck.com/mkgr/mmg/home.jsp>

Similar in format to the Merck Manual of Diagnosis and Therapy, this guide focuses on disorders and diseases with a slant towards implications for the elderly.

Merck Manual of Medical Information - 2nd Home Edition
<http://www.merck.com/mmhe/index.html>

A consumers' guide to diseases and their treatments. This is a complete online version of the text edition, with videos and a pronunciation guide

Postgraduate Medicine
<http://www.postgradmed.com/>
Professional medical journal with review articles on diseases and treatments. Although this is directed to the professional, the journal includes patient notes which are directed toward the general consumer.

MEDLINE/MedlinePlus
<http://www.nlm.nih.gov/medlineplus/>

Anatomy videos aimed at the general consumer plus thousands of articles on a variety of health related topics.

PubMed
<http://www.ncbi.nlm.nih.gov/sites/entrez>
PubMed comprises more than 20 million citations for biomedical literature from MEDLINE, life science journals, and online books. Citations may include links to full-text content from PubMed Central and publisher web sites.

News Services
These sources offer reliable information and up to date news stories about medical research.

Understanding Medical News

Consumer's Guide to Taking Charge of Medical Information
<http://www.health-insight-harvard.org/>

This guide, developed by the Harvard School of Public Health, helps you to decipher "scary" headlines.

Deciphering Medspeak
<http://mlanet.org/resources/medspeak/index.html>

To make informed health decisions, you have probably read a newspaper or magazine article, tuned into a radio or television program, or searched the Internet to find answers to health questions. If so, you have probably encountered "medspeak," the specialized language of health professionals. The Medical Library Association developed "Deciphering Medspeak" to help translate common "medspeak" terms.

HealthNewsReviews
<http://www.healthnewsreview.org/>
HealthNewsReview.org is a website dedicated to:
- Improving the accuracy of news stories about medical treatments, tests, products and procedures.
- Helping consumers evaluate the evidence for and against new ideas in health care.

Interpreting News on Diet and Nutrition
<http://www.hsph.harvard.edu/nutritionsource/nutrition-news/media/>

Confused by all the conflicting stories about what's good to eat and what's not? Sensational headlines don't always tell the whole story. Look at how nutrition news fits into the bigger scientific picture.

.

Understanding Risk. What Do Those Headlines Really Mean?
<http://www.niapublications.org/tipsheets/pdf/Understanding_Risk-What_Do_Those_Headlines_Really_Mean.pdf>

Tipsheet that discusses the differences among types of clinical research and explains the significance of types of risk in research results. Excellent easy to understand information about risk.

Beyond the Headlines: What Consumers Need To Know About Nutrition News
<http://www.foodinsight.org/>

The International Food Information Council Foundation is dedicated to the mission of effectively communicating science-based information on health, food safety and nutrition for the public good.

Recommended Online News Sources

Aetna InteliHealth Health News
<http://www.intelihealth.com/IH/ihtIH/WSIHW000/333/333.html?k=menux408x333>

Top news headlines for the day. There is a section with commentaries written by Harvard Medical School physicians of several of the day's top news stories.

CNN Health
<http://www.cnn.com/HEALTH/>

Daily updated articles from a variety of news sources with links to related CNN stories and websites.

1st Headlines - Top Health Headlines
<http://www.1stheadlines.com/health.htm>

Top news stories from a variety of sources. Story may be covered by more than one news sources, allowing you to compare stories and fill in information gaps.

Reuters Health eLine
<http://www.reutershealth.com/en/index.html>

Daily medical news for the consumer (free) and for the professional (requires a subscription fee).

News Sources with Daily or Weekly Email Delivery

MedlinePlus Health News
<http://www.nlm.nih.gov/medlineplus/>

Produced by the National Library of Medicine, this site has daily news releases from sources such as United Press International, New York Times Syndicate, and Reuters. Stories can be retrieved for thirty days from publication. Users may sign up for daily email of "Health Headlines" in several different categories.

Medscape
<http://www.medscape.com/>

From WebMD, a website for doctors with a comprehensive news feature. Go to the website to read the daily news or sign up for any of the forty free newsletters for delivery to your email address. There are newsletters in twenty-five specialties, a weekly multi-specialty edition, health business news, and much more.

NewsWise
<http://feeds.feedburner.com/NewswiseMednews>
Medical news stories. Information from news releases of more than four hundred universities, professional associations, and research institutions. Register and sign up to receive weekly medical news digests via email.

Alternative Medicine Ask Dr. Weil
<http://www.drweil.com/>

The popular doctor discusses alternative healing remedies for many common ailments.

Alternative Medicine Homepage
<http://www.pitt.edu/~cbw/altm.html>
From the Falk Library of the Health Sciences, University of Pittsburgh - a jumpstation for sources of information on unconventional, alternative, complementary, innovative, and integrative therapies.

HerbMed

<http://www.herbmed.org/>

HerbMed is an interactive, electronic herbal database. It provides hyperlinked access to the scientific & medical research articles on the use of herbs for treating medical conditions. This evidence-based information resource is for professionals, researchers, and the general public.

National Center for Complementary and Alternative Medicine
<http://nccam.nih.gov/>

General information about alternative and complementary therapies with links to research studies currently being conducted on alternative therapies for a variety of conditions.

Rosenthal Center for Complementary and Alternative Medicine
<http://www.rosenthal.hs.columbia.edu//>

Links to resources on acupuncture, homeopathy, chiropractic, and herbal medicine and alternative therapies for cancer and women's health. The Center sponsors research on alternative and complementary medical practices.

Clinical Research Trials

Center Watch
<http://www.centerwatch.com/>

Information on over 41,000 clinical trials for twenty disease categories. Profiles of 150 research centers conducting clinical trials and profiles of companies that provide a variety of contract services to the clinical trials industry. Includes industry and government sponsored clinical trials and information on new drug treatments approved by the Food and Drug Administration.

Clinical Trials
<http://www.clinicaltrials.gov/>

Information on current research being conducted on treatments for different diseases. Browse by disease category and sponsor or search the entire site. Learn what clinical trials are all about and how to decide to participate in a trial.

Diseases, Medical Conditions, General Health

Aetna Intelihealth
<http://www.intelihealth.com/IH/ihtIH?t=408>

From the Harvard Medical School, information on diseases and medical conditions, health and fitness, medications, nutrition, childbirth, and other topics.

Healthfinder
<http://www.healthfinder.gov/>

From the U.S. Department of Health and Human Services, a gateway to consumer information on diseases, medical conditions, health promotion, and many other topics.

Mayo Clinic

<http://www.mayoclinic.com/>

From the famed Mayo Clinic, information on diseases and conditions, treatment decisions, drugs and supplements, healthy living, and health assessment tools. Special features include online videos of exercises, diagnostic tests, surgical procedures, and medical conditions, healthy recipes, and self-care information.

National Organization for Rare Diseases

<http://www.rarediseases.org/>

Basic information on rare diseases and disorders. Full-reports are available for a fee.

NOAH (New York Online Access to Health)
<http://www.noah-health.org/>
English and Spanish language information and resources from organizations and governmental agencies. Aging, cancer, asthma, eye diseases, foot and ankle disorders, and pain are just a few of the topics covered.

Health Care Providers

American Board of Medical Specialties (ABMS)
<http://www.abms.org/>

Verify the certification status of any physician in the 24 specialities of the ABMS. Registration is required (free) and user is limited to five searches in a 24 hour period.

AMA Physician Select
<https://extapps.ama-assn.org/doctorfinder/recaptcha.jsp>

Gives credentials of MD's and DO's including medical school, year of graduation, and specialties.

American Hospital Directory
<http://www.ahd.com/>
Profiles of U.S. hospitals. Basic service is free; more detailed information by paid subscription only.

Federation of State Medical Boards
<http://www.fsmb.org/>

Select "Public Services" from the left-hand index, then select "Directory of State Medical Boards" to find links to web sites for the 50 U.S. States, plus the District of Columbia, Guam, and the Northern Mariana Islands. Not all of the states have physician profile or disciplinary action information. There are also links to osteopathic physician sites when available.

Health Pages
<http://www.healthpages.com/>

Information about physicians, dentists, hospitals and clinics, elder care facilities, dietitians and nutritionists.

Joint Commission on the Accreditation of Healthcare Organizations
<http://www.jointcommission.org/>
The Quality Check feature on this site supplies details on individual hospital performance ratings from JCAHO's accreditation reports. View Performance Reports and compare institutions' ratings. Reports cover hospitals, nursing homes, ambulatory care facilities, home care, laboratory

services, and long term care facilities.

Nursing Home Compare
<http://www.medicare.gov/NHCompare/Include/DataSection/Questions/SearchCriteriaNEW.asp?version=default&browser=Chrome|6|WinNT&language=English&defaultstatus=0&pagelist=Home&CookiesEnabledStatus=True>
Provides detailed information about the performance of every Medicare and Medicaid certified nursing home in the country. Searchable by state. Includes a guide to choosing a nursing home and a nursing home checklist to help in making informed choices.

Questions and Answers about Health Insurance: A Consumer Guide

<http://www.ahrq.gov/consumer/insuranceqa/>

Questions and answers on choosing and using a health plan.

Quackery and Health Fraud

Quackwatch
<http://www.quackwatch.com/>

Want information about whether those alternative therapies work? This site has information on health fraud, medical quackery, "new age" medicine and "alternative" and "complementary" medicine.

National Council against Health Fraud
<http://www.ncahf.org/>
Non-profit voluntary health agency focusing on health fraud,

misinformation, and quackery as public health oncerns. Read their position papers on acupuncture, homepathy, chiropractic, and other health issues.

Surgery

American College of Surgeons
<http://www.facs.org/>
   Public information section offers guidelines on choosing a qualified surgeon.

Tests and Procedures - MedlinePlus

<http://www.nlm.nih.gov/medlineplus/tutorial.html   >
Interactive tutorials on 24 common tests and diagnostic procedures and more than 30 surgeries and treatment procedures.

Manufactured by Amazon.ca
Bolton, ON